Paul Valent is an internationally renowned traumatologist with a background in medicine, psychiatry, and psychotherapy. Influenced by his Holocaust experiences as a child, he was always interested in trauma. He was liaison psychiatrist in the Monash Medical Centre emergency department in Melbourne for 25 years, where he treated many traumatised patients. He initiated a mental health team in the Ash Wednesday bushfires.

Valent founded the Melbourne Child Survivors of the Holocaust group and cofounded the Australasian Society for Traumatic Stress Studies. He presided over the 2000 International Society for Traumatic Stress Studies World Conference.

His publications include numerous papers, encyclopaedia entries and lectures. His first book was *Child Survivors of the Holocaust: Adults Living with Childhood Trauma*. His *From Survival to Fulfilment: A Framework for the Life-Trauma Dialectic* and *Trauma and Fulfilment Therapy: A Wholist Framework* are pioneering texts in traumatology. *In Two Minds: Tales of a Psychotherapist* and his latest book, *Heart of Violence: Why People Harm Each Other,* are suitable for both professionals and the general public.

MENTAL HEALTH

IN THE TIMES
OF THE

PANDEMIC

PAUL VALENT

Australian Scholarly

First published 2020 by
Australian Scholarly Publishing Ltd
7 Lt Lothian St Nth, North Melbourne, Vic 3051
Tel: 03 9329 6963 / Fax: 03 9329 5452
enquiry@scholarly.info / www.scholarly.info

ISBN 978-1-922454-05-8

Cover design: Wayne Saunders

To Dani, Ariel and Amy

Contents

Acknowledgements

I am very grateful to the following, who unhesitatingly and unstintingly provided me of their experiences and wisdom: Prof Grant Blashki, Michael Breen, Prof Tony Guttmann, Rana Hussain, Amelia Klein, Prof Pat McGorry, Dr Natasha Rabbidge, Sr Natasha Reisner, James Walker, Ted Watts.

I have also referred to 4 Corners ABC/PBS and to publications by the Red Cross, Beyondblue and Emergency Management Australia.

Special acknowledgement to Nick Walker, who inspired this book, and the staff of Australian Scholarly Publishing who produced it.

Preface

'My mind is racing about this crisis.' 'It's just like a flu, really. Only 3% die.' 'Is the person who handled my food infected?' 'We'll beat this!' 'I am a nurse, I care and care. I come home and I care. I am weary and worn out with caring.' 'We're all in this together, but I feel alone.' 'Will people see me queuing for food?' 'I have to sack people who've been like family.' 'I roller coaster from anger, fear, and crying to total numbness.' 'My chest is lead.' 'My chest is painful.' 'My chest is exploding.' 'My mummy is angry.' 'I feel honoured to be able to help on the frontline.'

These are just a few comments shared during the COVID–19 (Corona virus disease 2019) pandemic. They are a sample of what is referred to as the increasing mental health consequences of the pandemic.

Often mental health effects of the pandemic are said to be anxiety, depression, and suicidal ideas. But our small sample indicates that mental health effects are widespread and cannot be encapsulated in a few words.

The pandemic threw our world up in the air. We deal with the immediacy of survival. We try to orientate ourselves, but our minds are in a fog. We are captured by the many feelings and sensations sampled above.

We try to take control even as we are preoccupied with our personal, family, work, economic, political, and yes, even spiritual challenges.

We try to make sense of this in terms of other crises. Is this a disaster, like the recent bushfires? Or like a war, with which many people compare the pandemic. Are we hiding in the trenches while we wait for weapons (vaccine) that will lead us to victory? Or is this like the Great Depression, with so many unemployed and people going bankrupt.

Lastly, we wonder when and how all this will end, and what will be beyond? Will we be confronted by a cascade of disruptions, fragmented structures and enmities, or will our better natures emerge? Will we have learned new means, created new horizons? Come to see the world differently, and harness revived purpose to other challenges? Could that be the silver lining in this pandemic?

Luckily, since the last major pandemic, the 1918 Spanish flu, we have developed much knowledge about disaster responses.

Knowledge of human responses in disasters can help individuals and societies to understand themselves better and hence to control better their presents and futures.

The purpose of this book is to help orientate and make sense of the very wide mental health effects of this pandemic, and thereby to help assuage distress and fashion a better future.

Following the Introduction in chapter 1, I present in chapter 2 a summary of ubiquitous disaster responses, as they have manifested in this pandemic. The responses are divided into biological, psychological and social ones, as they occur in individuals, families, children and vulnerable groups. The chapter offers some helpful do's and don'ts. This chapter is an expanded version of a pamphlet *How to Cope With a Major Personal Crisis* that has been distributed in Australian and overseas disasters for over three decades.

Chapter 3 provides a framework which helps to orientate, understand and treat the wide-ranging consequences of the pandemic.

Because major crises evoke not only efforts to survive, but also reveal the range of human aspirations, we learn through our responses not only about human vulnerabilities but also about our potentials and fulfilments.

This book is suitable for both professionals and the interested public. Chapter 2 is suitable for general readership. The pamphlet on which it is based has been shown to be widely accessible and helpful.

1.

INTRODUCTION

All threats to life appear to be unique to those experiencing them. And yet, from a different vantage point, all threats share commonalities. For instance, each event has a lead-up time, a time of striking, a time of reeling and a time of recovery. Scientific terms for these times are pre-impact phase, impact phase, post-impact phase, and recovery phase.

Similarly, each situation involves individuals, families, groups and communities; adults and children; the fit and the vulnerable; leaders and followers.

Each situation is physically, emotionally and socially stressful, and in each a certain set of inherited stress responses attempt to restore equilibrium.

Though all traumatic situations share commonalities, they are also different. We sense that car accidents differ from floods, and both differ from wars.

It is here that we try to orientate the pandemic, a disaster or traumatic situation outside our prior experience.

Let's see what we know of past epidemics and pandemics.

Past Epidemics and Pandemics

Widespread epidemics have occurred throughout history. In the Plague of Athens in 430BC Athenians lost 100,000 people. This was miniscule compared to the Antonine Plague AD165–80, which laid waste the Roman army and killed five million people, not counting the invasions and civil wars that followed.

Similarly, the Plague of Justinian 541–42, which might have wiped out 10% of the world's population, saw the gradual demise of the Byzantine Empire.

The Black Death or Plague of 1346–53 is estimated to have wiped out 25 million people, a third to a half of Europe's population.

The American plagues of the 16th century, introduced by Europeans, killed off 90% of the Aztec, Inca, and American Indian civilisations, facilitating European conquest of the Western hemisphere.

The Spanish flu pandemic of 1918–20 infected around 500 million people or one-third of the world's population. It claimed at least 50 million deaths. The poor conditions of soldiers fighting World War I enhanced the spread and lethality of the virus.

In recent times the Asian flu 1957–58 killed a million people, mainly in Singapore and Hong Kong. The AIDS pandemic, which broke out in 1981 has killed 35 million people around the world. Around 40 million are still infected with it, but medication is allowing them to live normal lives. Lastly, the 2009 H1N1 swine-flu pandemic killed up to half a million people. A vaccine against this flu is included with regular flu vaccines.

The Current Pandemic

Origin. SARSCoV–2, generally referred to as Covid–19 (Corona virus disease 2019) appears to have originated in the Huanan seafood wholesale wet market in Wuhan, China in late 2019. The virus was probably transmitted from bat corona viruses. By March 2020 the virus spread around the world sufficiently for the WHO to declare a pandemic.

Prevalence. By September 2020 over 25 million cases and over 800,000 deaths due to Covid–19 were reported around the world.

Because many infected people do not reveal symptoms or only have mild symptoms, and because in many cases statistics are unreliable, the proportion of severe and lethal infections out of total infections is unknown. However, it is estimated that around 1% of all those infected die. Those with significant symptoms have a higher, 1–10%, chance of dying.

Rates of infection and mortality are influenced by many factors. Throughout the world relatively high rates of infection were more likely in situations of poverty, overcrowding, lack of education, and need to take on risky jobs where infections were more likely. Associated with their social disadvantages, in America African-Americans died at three times the rate of white Americans.

Death rates increased with age, especially if the old had underlying medical conditions. The initial high death rates in Italy, which overwhelmed the health services, were attributed to a relatively old population. Aged care homes poorly served by untrained casual staff were responsible for a second wave of infection in Melbourne, which resulted in hundreds of deaths.

No vulnerable part of the community can be ignored. For instance, having coped well with the first wave of the virus, Singapore and Thailand suffered second waves that started in ignored, overcrowded pockets of migrant populations.

One special group at risk comprised health care workers. By April 2020 approximately 200 doctors had died of corona virus around the world. By June, 898 health care workers died in the USA alone. By August it was estimated that 10% of corona treating health care workers in different parts of the world had been infected. The attrition of staff added to the stress of the remaining workers.

Having said all this, the greatest influence on the prevalence of the disease is the approach to it by the national leaders. South Korea and Singapore, with previous experience of epidemics were quick to impose stringent hygiene and isolation measures and their populations were relatively spared, even with the second wave. England took time to acknowledge the seriousness of the pandemic. Sweden chose herd immunity and let the pandemic rip. Brazil took a macho, indifferent attitude, and in the USA president Trump scoffed at the disease as a Democratic Party hoax. The latter countries, especially the USA (over 200,000 deaths), have suffered severe infection and mortality rates.

Realistic appraisals and actions were the best protection against the disease.

Symptoms. According to the WHO, symptoms arise one to fourteen days after contraction of the disease. The commonest symptoms are fever, dry cough, and fatigue. Less common are sputum, loss of taste and smell, shortness of breath, muscle and joint pains, sore throat, headaches, chills, vomiting, coughing blood, diarrhoea and rash, and depression and anxiety. Other long-term effects are being investigated.

Treatment. The best treatment is prevention, but this requires a vaccine which to date is not available.

Most infections are not severe, and treatment is symptomatic, meaning treatment is directed to alleviate specific symptoms. For instance, ventilators help to provide oxygen to those with severe lung infections.

Once inside a population, eradication of the virus is difficult. Various techniques, however, suppress spread of the virus: closing borders, quarantining arrivals, screening of the population and quarantining infected people and their contacts, social distancing, lockdown of inessential businesses, schools and workers, isolation of populations in their homes, wearing of masks, hand washing and frequent sanitisation.

All these measures help prevent the spread of infections, prevent health services from being overwhelmed, and provide time for new treatments and development of a vaccine.

Prognosis depends on success of preventive measures, efficacy of the political and health systems, dealing with further outbreaks and 'second waves', but especially on availability of a vaccine. Once infected, most people survive, depending on the severity of the disease and available help. However, some symptoms can linger or return.

Secondary consequences. Disruptions of individual, family, work, community, and international systems and relationships have a variety of detrimental consequences.

Suicides, domestic violence, accidents, and a variety of illnesses may increase as in other disasters. So far domestic violence has manifested most overtly. Nevertheless, social splits and blames, us-them boundaries, and societal, racial, and xenophobic tendencies have emerged around the world. Some say that secondary economic, health, social, and political consequences may be more damaging than the virus.

Secondary consequences are widespread. In the absence of a vaccine the pandemic could rumble on for years. It has already caused strains on health services, havoc with economies, and political tensions. It has caused widespread mental health deterioration, ranging from individuals to nations.

In summary, like the spread of the physical virus, expanding concentric circles of its effects manifest physically, psychologically, and socially from individuals to nations.

2.

EXPERIENCING AND COPING WITH THE PANDEMIC

This chapter names and provides words to frequently unnamed and unthought experiences. Words crystallise such experiences and provide means to think about, understand and deal with them. Understanding one's internal environment can be as useful as understanding one's external environment.

Mental health issues have been becoming ever more prominent in this pandemic, as they do during other disasters. However, psychiatric illnesses increase only a little. Most mental health issues, even the usually recognised anxiety, depression, and suicide rates, can be best understood in terms of a wide range of stress and trauma responses rather than as psychiatric illnesses.

Nevertheless, psychiatric illnesses do flare up or deteriorate when the pandemic strikes at previous vulnerabilities that had caused those illnesses in the past.

What follows are thumbnail descriptions of common mental, physical, and social (biopsychosocial) responses to disasters as manifested in this pandemic. Understanding these responses can lead to better means of mitigating them.

As mentioned, this chapter is an expanded version of a pamphlet *How to Cope With a Major Personal Crisis* that has been distributed in Australian and overseas disasters for over three decades.

CONSEQUENCES OF PANDEMIC STRESS

The responses below apply to responses to the pandemic as well as to its secondary consequences such as bereavement and unemployment.

Feelings and Emotions Commonly Felt in the Pandemic

Shock and Disbelief. Initially the pandemic felt unreal, like a dream or a film. The invisibility of the virus and the small number of people initially affected facilitated denial. 'Perhaps it will only be like a bad flu.'

Fear and Anxiety has been the other side of disbelief. Fears included: the virus will kill me, 'eat me up', or my family; I will be left alone; abandoned; betrayed; I may fail in my duties; I may do something that will harm others. Anxiety may verge on panic.

Helplessness and Powerlessness are accentuated by the pervasiveness and invisibility of the virus.

Dependence. People depend on authorities for information, guidance, and hope. They willingly give up freedoms they previously fought hard to preserve and obey new constricting rules. Some make a show of their independence and flout the rules.

Loneliness and Longing for family and friends whom one cannot see and touch. Yearning for all that has gone, some things perhaps forever.

Sadness, Grief and Depression following bereavements, illnesses, and losses of all kinds.

Despair when the pandemic drags on, second waves appear, consequences keep escalating, and no end seems in sight.

Anger with leaders who do not care, who have been remiss. Frustration and impotence due to inability to proceed with one's life. Outrage with the senselessness and injustice of it all. Anger with 'others', and scapegoats for one's suffering.

Guilt for being alive and healthy, for being better off than others, for failing to save or help others, for not preventing one's children from suffering.

Shame for being helpless, dependent, emotional; for being passive, cowardly.

Over-Immersion and Over-Arousal. People may follow every detail of the pandemic. This may alternate with

Numbness when people cut themselves off from information and feelings. Feelings may rumble below, and surface unexpectedly.

Let-Downs and disappointments, for instance with recurrent waves of the virus, which may alternate with

Hope for the future and better times, especially as infections and death rates decrease.

All these feelings can occur individually or in combinations. They can occur in relation to the virus itself, or in relation to secondary stresses such as unemployment, or not being able to pay the rent.

The feelings are common and normal, and allowing their expression leads not to loss of control as may be feared, but to relief and healing. **Bottling up feelings can lead to nervous and physical problems.**

Perceptual and Physical Responses

Time may drag with boredom, yet in retrospect to have flown by.

Memory and concentration. One's mind may become fuzzy and constricted.

Fatigue may ensue from sleeplessness, constant vigilance, and need to reassess what were everyday automatic activities.

Common physical symptoms include dizziness, palpitations, shakes, choking in the throat, nausea, diarrhoea, and pains in the head, neck, chest and back. Women may experience dragging in the womb and menstrual disorders. Either gender may experience changes in sexual interest.

Secondary physical effects. Infections, hypertension, cardiac disease, diabetes, and other illnesses may arise from or be aggravated by stress.

Increased intakes of coffee, alcohol and drugs has occurred. Some people abandoned their treatment regimes. Some took up gambling.

Accidents—stress leads to increases in domestic, car, motorbike and bicycle accidents.

Paradoxical improvements can result from lockdowns, such as fewer infections due to less social mixing.

Family and Social Relationships

The pandemic has produced different and even opposing consequences depending on prevailing circumstances. For instance, separations from family members due to closed borders and lockdowns was hard to bear, but in other circumstances close and prolonged proximity could fray the nerves. Similarly, enforced closeness increased intimacy in many families, while it led to domestic violence in others.

The same applied to work. Working from home, with children doing simultaneous home schooling and making other demands, often stretched the nerves. On the other hand, not having to travel to work and not be distracted by fellow workers could improve productivity.

Increased leisure time could be enjoyable but being unemployed and bereft of social activities could be stressful. Zoom meetings were a compensation, but they could become sterile, and frustrating due to technological difficulties.

In the wider community, 'We are alone together' expressed solidarity, but this was not enhanced by social distancing and lockdowns. Inevitably, suspicions arose of others carrying the virus. A tendency toward us-them delineations emerged, ranging from individuals and neighbourhoods to between states and nations.

Authorities that cared, were truthful and communicated clearly were trusted and obeyed. Leaders who were self-focused, denied the truth, were incompetent and offered false hope, even as the mortality rates grew, evoked anger and a sense of betrayal among their citizens.

People who mistrusted authorities from past experience could interpret lockdowns as being imprisoned, picked on or unjustly punished. They could rebel, protest, and even be violent.

Children

Though adults put themselves out and sacrificed their own needs for their children, they were often impervious to the children's own distress. Attention to children's feelings could add to the stress of already burdened parents.

Children responded similarly to adults, except that their responses were shaped by their age, imagination, dependence on adults, and maturity of understanding. Children feared especially the loss of their parents, family, and friends. They were especially worried, too, that their actions could damage their parents or cause their loss.

During lockdowns children missed their schools, learning, friends, teachers and routines. Paradoxically, some children who previously did not mix well with others thrived through distant learning.

Being less able to express themselves verbally, children may express themselves through behaviour. They may sleep poorly, have nightmares, regress and be clingier, bed wet again, withdraw, or they may become disruptive.

Vulnerable Groups

The Elderly are more vulnerable to the virus, especially if they have underlying disabilities, illnesses, dementia, and if they are in nursing homes where the virus can spread easily. All these circumstances add to the vulnerability of their mental health.

The Ill, whether from the corona virus or other illnesses, are susceptible to mental health problems. They increase due to forced separation from families during lockdowns.

The Bereaved. To normal grief is added pain of having been prevented to be with the dying, and funeral services being severely scaled back.

The Socially Isolated suffer extra aloneness and vulnerability. Those stuck in foreign countries, migrants who cannot understand the local language, and those unable to use electronic media suffer extra isolation and lack of support.

The Already Stressed and Traumatised. The pandemic may add to prior stresses such as poverty and illnesses. The poor live in more crowded situations and find it harder to isolate and not work. They may ignore corona symptoms because they may not have food if they don't work. In addition, current stresses may add to and trigger old traumas.

HELPERS give deeply of themselves. They anguish over their clients and patients and are prone to feel guilt for not having done enough for them. They are haunted by their patients' deaths, and distraught by the possibility of having to choose who would be treated and who left to die. Overwork, lack of sleep, lack of resources and emotional buffeting lead them to exhaustion and 'burn-out'.

Helpers worry about transmitting the virus to other patients and to their families. Only secondarily do they worry about being infected themselves. Many helpers in fact have become infected, and quite a few, such as in Italy, have died. Attrition of staff through illness and quarantine increases stress on the rest.

Cascades of Stress

Previous stresses and stress responses can accumulate in various combinations with new stresses and produce cascades of stress and trauma. For instance, in parts of the USA the virus was the last straw on top of unemployment, poor housing, racial tensions, police brutality and poverty. In the end the situation exploded in riots and violence.

In the USA, too, the virus became embroiled in local political division and in international tension.

Making the Event Easier To Bear

Mental Defences. Initially the severity of the pandemic was denied and downplayed before it was finally accepted. However, some kept on denying the facts, and a few devised conspiracy theories about malign powers taking away their rights. Denial beyond what was needed to absorb the shock led to danger to self and others.

Reality and facts though painful initially, provide best value in the long run. They forestall myths and fantasies that may increase distress and danger. It was therefore important to stick to a narrow range of trustworthy information.

Expression of Feelings. Allowing feelings to surface and

expressing them provides relief and control, not loss of control, as is often feared.

Support can provide great relief and comfort. Mutual support can foster camaraderie and friendship.

Useful activity such as working online, helping others, setting up games for children provide a sense of control and normality.

Routines provide a sense of constancy and reality.

Humour, *music*, *films*, provide perspective and relief.

Privacy is important even in isolation. It allows digestion of feelings and contextualisation of oneself in the world.

Hope. Remembering pre-pandemic pasts and prospects of post-pandemic futures puts the pandemic in context. There will be an end to the pandemic. Wounds will heal. We may even come out of this disaster stronger and wiser.

Silver Linings

It's said that every cloud has a silver lining, and the pandemic threw up a few disparate ones.

Helpers derived deep satisfaction from saving and maintaining lives and essential comforts of others. They did not feel heroic, but they understood that they were at the forefront of historical events.

In the population, especially initially, unprecedented cooperation arose among previously separate social groups. 'We are alone but in this together' this time signified the paradox of social isolation shared throughout populations.

Many adjusted to new realities. People became technology savvy. People used the internet for work, schooling, individual, family, and group meetings and games. The internet provided connections and entertainment from around the world.

Work and study at home saved travel time and provided extra time for hobbies, intimate relationships and thinking.

Stripped of inessentials, people had the chance to learn about themselves, and who and what was important in their lives.

Cobwebs of old thinking may be swept away to be replaced by wisdom, pragmatism, creativity and cooperation. Realistic perspectives may be reinforced and be translated into action, such as on climate change and economic inequalities.

Some Do's

DO follow Government and Health Department guidelines.

DO try to be realistic in terms of the world and yourself.

DO express your needs and feelings and encourage those around you, especially children, to do the same. Help young children to express themselves in drawings and play.

DO establish routines of work, exercise, study, and hobbies.

DO take time out to sleep, rest, think, enjoy and be intimate.

DO be more careful around your home and work.

DO drive more carefully.

DO maintain your medications.

DO be careful with your intake of food, alcohol, and drugs.

DO seek professional help when unwell or overwhelmed.

REMEMBER that you are the same person as you were before the pandemic.

REMEMBER that there is light at the end of the tunnel.

3.

ORIENTATION AND UNDERSTANDING MENTAL HEALTH CONSEQUENCES OF THE PANDEMIC

In the last chapter we noted common responses in disasters and their particular manifestations in the pandemic. What has been missing are actual pandemic stories and a framework for understanding their complexities.

Complexity of the Pandemic

We need to understand first that there are complexities. It is not simply fear of death, of ourselves and our loved ones, and that's it. To explain what I mean, let's take a simple example of one's world being thrown up in the air. Let us use a simple analogy of a car crash.

Even here many questions arise. What were the driving conditions like? What about the car: brakes, steering, and so on? Then innumerable questions about the driver. Age, gender, experience, state of sobriety, drug intake, personality such as general aggressiveness, previous accidents; stresses that could have influenced appraisals of the situation—distractions for instance due to recent grief;

and then motivations, perhaps even suicidal intentions? And we can compare this incident with general statistics: frequency of crashes among the young, the old, men and women, the inebriated and drugged, in cities and countryside, in different countries, and so on.

Then come the many questions regarding consequences. How was the driver affected, when, and how? Did the driver suffer recurrent fears, nightmares, helplessness, grief, anger, guilt? What secondary stresses occurred- in hospital, with insurance companies, without transport? And what did this mean in the person's life and to those around?

It appears that the questions are endless. Yet all are important and dispensing with any of them leaves important questions unresolved.

In the previous chapter some organization of these questions was already apparent. Experiences were classified according to biological, psychological, and social responses, in children and adults, and in individuals and communities.

Compared to a car crash the pandemic 'crash' is so widespread and complex that one may think that it is impossible to contain its myriad fragments in a coherent body of knowledge.

In the physical world we have myriads of experiences, such as gravity and energy, which can be named and captured in mathematical formulae. Perhaps experiences of survival may be similarly tethered to a formula of sorts.

Right now, we are *experiencing* the pandemic, just as we are experiencing gravity or energy. I will try to describe the experiences of the pandemic while tethering them to a scientific whole. I call this the wholist perspective. To pre-empt, the wholist perspective consists of eight survival drives in three dimensions.

The wholist perspective is applicable across human crises and catastrophes. It has been applied in individual crises, community disasters, and it is applicable to future looming crises.

Let me give a thumbnail description of the pandemic as seen from mid to late 2020. My situation is Melbourne, Australia, which is in Stage 4 lockdown following a second wave of the virus. First and second waves of the pandemic are currently being experienced in different parts of the world.

EARLY APPRAISALS OF AND RESPONSES TO THE PANDEMIC

Leaders

Denial of approaching disasters was common, as acknowledgement carried great costs. Warnings by Chinese doctors of the threat of a new lethal virus were officially denied and suppressed for up to two months.

Eventually heavy isolation measures were imposed, and the virus was suppressed.

In the USA, the pandemic did not suit President Trump. He called the pandemic an ordinary flu, a Democratic Party beat-up and fake news. Later, he blamed China, the WHO and the 'radical' left for the spread of the virus. The nation divided along political lines. Half the population followed Trump's anti-factual stance and dispensed with appropriate precautions. The result was that a quarter of the world's pandemic deaths consisted of Americans, and the numbers are still rising.

Brazil's president Bolsonaro's macho denial, UK's Boris Johnson's erratic attitude, and Sweden's calculated choice of letting the virus rip till herd immunity was achieved, all led to high infection rates in their countries, and, incidentally, in the cases of Bolsonaro, Johnson and Trump, to their own infections.

South Korea, Singapore, New Zealand and Australia had relatively low infection rates due to their geographic isolation, united governments, respect for science, and early social distancing measures. Nevertheless, second waves, as we saw, remained a threat.

In summary, leaders who did not face the realities of the pandemic risked the lives of their citizens. Leaders who provided unambiguous, factual, credible and purposeful messages were believed and their warnings were heeded to the benefit of their populations.

Populations

Populations were influenced by attitudes of their leaders, by their own propensities, and by the nature of the pandemic.

The invisibility of the virus and initial distance from it favoured denial, and a sense of a distant cloud that may pass one by. As the pandemic became more real, people bargained: 'Perhaps it is just a more severe flu.' 'Perhaps only the old and sick will die.' Some blamed the messenger or rebelled against the message: 'Perhaps they are wrong.' 'Perhaps the government is using the pandemic to take away our freedoms.'

As the death rates climbed, reality started to penetrate. Populations accepted the facts and complied with restrictions.

Still, denial and rebellion persisted to varying degrees. They could lead to a sense of euphoria, a macho type victory. For instance, a man in Texas attended a 'Covid party' to demonstrate that the virus was not real. Before he died, he said, 'I thought this was a hoax, but it's not.'

Some attended religious services in the belief that God would protect them. The congregations became infection 'hot spots'.

In the USA and Germany groups protested in the streets against restrictions of their democratic rights to congregate, to move freely, and to breathe freely without masks. The protests were reminiscent of past protests against fluoridation of water supplies.

People injected individual problems, agendas, and conspiracy theories into the protests. A man with sadistic tendencies refused to wear a mask. He enjoyed the discomfort of those around him.

As most populations accepted the necessity of the strictures and obeyed orders of hygiene, alertness, isolation, and social distancing, they felt that they were slipping into a different world, which another part of their minds found difficult to absorb.

Like Alice in Wonderland, the world and one's self were unreal, topsy-turvy. For instance, people were told that to fight the enemy they were to do nothing. They should not work, and the government would pay them for that. Governments for whom debt was anathema, injected many billions of debt into the economy. Everyday life somersaulted. Forbidden behaviours were going out, meeting friends and relatives, even touching and hugging.

People absorbed the situation in fragments. One way was through humour, irony, and sarcasm. Jokes and cartoons abounded, such as of a woman standing in front of her wardrobe, bemoaning the fact that she now had to add her mask into the mix of trying to coordinate her dress. Referring to a run on toilet paper, a girl asks her father sitting on a throne of toilet rolls, 'Daddy, what did you do in the war?' A young child made up a rap song, 'Boo, Coronavirus'.

Fear and other emotions broke through the barriers, as

noted in the Preface. A woman wrote on Twitter, 'Feeling very anxious this morning ... hearing about further lockdowns. It's a feeling of terror actually, heart racing, hot, teary. There is no tiger about to attack me but it sure feels that way.'

A doctor rostered soon for a corona ward felt as if a tsunami was approaching. 'Would I come out the other end after being submerged or would I be dumped?' Doctors were concerned at the lack of beds, equipment, and personal protective equipment. Would they become infected? Would they infect others?

At the Epicentre: A Patient and a Healer

So far most members of populations have not been infected by the virus. But many have been, and many health workers have been too.

Let us go to the epicentre of the problem—a patient, and a healer.

Tony, academic aged 75, Melbourne

Tony attended a conference in which a colleague from overseas showed him excitedly his new textbook. Tony leafed through it for a few minutes.

That evening the friend rang to say that he was unwell and had temperature. He tested positive for COVID. Tony, still unaffected the next day, ran two laps around the local lake. However, by the evening he felt 'fluey', had himself tested and isolated himself. 'I hope I won't die,' he thought. 'What a stupid way to die.'

The friend recovered after five days, and Tony also just felt like he had a mild flu. But then extreme fatigue set in. He slept, dreamless, 22 hours a day for two weeks. He could only eat soup and he lost 6 kilograms in weight.

Apart from rearranging his will, he had no interest in anything, though he did think, 'What a messy attic to leave to the children.'

Tony's brain felt 'fuzzy'. One night going to the toilet he became disoriented, fell, and lost consciousness for a few seconds. He fell again soon after, without losing consciousness.

After two weeks, Tony started to recover and gain strength. For some weeks he continued to have urinary and bowel symptoms, but they resolved too. He returned to the same fitness as he held before his infection.

The colleague continues to have waves of exhaustion.

Tony's wife felt 'depleted' for a couple of days at the beginning of Tony's illness, but suffered no more symptoms.

His experience brought Tony face to face with his mortality. He came to appreciate his family more than before. He was touched by the solicitude of his wife and neighbours. 'I became kinder, more tolerant, less arrogant. Much what I had considered important, I now see as peripheral.

'Love, connections, truth, and decency are more important.'

A view from the frontline: Cremona March 2020

In March 2020 Italy was one of the most highly corona infected countries. At the peak of the pandemic almost 1000 people died each day. Cremona was at the epicentre of the pandemic, and its hospital ICU (Intensive Care Unit) was at the core of the epicentre.

Initially the doctors were unconcerned at reports of the virus. They perceived it as far away. Then it threatened a nearby town. Then came the avalanche. PBS Frontline: Inside Italy's COVID WAR filmed the events.

Doctors worked 12-hour shifts. Patients waited for hours and hours. Laura, a doctor, said of the patients, 'I admire their capacity. They don't know their fate. [And we] have no answers.' Laura was on the brink of tears.

A patient aged 30 had resisted her husband's fear of her going to the hospital. 'I think I have early pneumonia … I hope, but I'm scared … It's a nightmare … The youngest, aged 3 can't do without me … I'm worried, sad.' She rings her husband and cries, 'I can't handle this. I'm scared.' She is diagnosed positive for the virus and is admitted.

The doctor is expressionless. 'It's an unfair battle. We have few weapons. The virus has them all. We fight anyway ... The worst is having to choose whom to intubate; who should have oxygen.'

At home Laura unburdens to her husband, who has supported her going to the hospital, 'We're dropping like flies.' Half the doctors are infected. Laura has not hugged her husband for a month for fear of infecting him. He has compromised lungs.

Mattia, aged 18 is brought in. His mother is devastated because she can't be close. Mother asks nurses to hold his hand. Mattia whispers, 'I'm scared I'm going to die.' Laura wants to throw herself at him, to protect him. 'All my heart, but ... damn it!' She is afraid of becoming infected herself, and even worse, she may infect her patients and her family.

The virus is circulating, getting closer. Laura is tired, worn out, scared. She becomes infected and goes into isolation at home. 'It's weird. I crossed to the other side.'

Her 13-year-old son tries to be brave. 'Mother will make it. She is like Captain America ... She does it for others.' Laura's 11-year-old daughter says, 'I just thought of her as a doctor. Now I'm scared she'll bring it home ... I'm afraid for father ... I'm proud of her.' She tries to hold back tears but can't. 'I'm scared for my parents..my brother and me left alone ... I don't know how to cook ... how to divide chores ... We don't know how to do anything.' She bursts into sobs.

The son leaves food outside Laura's room. 'Thank you for your company,' she says sarcastically. Lack of physical contact is driving her crazy. 'Do you miss my scolding?' They laugh.

She is fatigued, feels useless, cries. Yells to a colleague 'visiting her' in the street, 'I feel like jumping out the window.' 'No, you're too low to kill yourself. And think of the damage to the pavement.' They laugh.

Laura recovers. Back in the ward, so does Mattia. He raises everyone's morale. 'You are our victory.' It felt like a rebirth among so much death.

After three months of avoiding touching, the staff hug each other. They are united in their desire to grab and enjoy life. They feel sad for those who couldn't make it.

A second wave of the pandemic arrives.

Let us now move away from the epicentre.

Ripples of the Pandemic

Ripples from the pandemic varied greatly. Many in the population adapted to working and studying from home and enjoyed being with family. But they were strained trying to juggle multiple jobs, supervising children, and keeping up with household requirements.

The internet was enlisted to help overcome isolation,

disconnections from work, school, and society. Many arranged regular internet family meetings, book, exercise and hobby groups, and 'play dates' among children. But lack of closeness and artificiality of the media made the meetings less genuine and useful. Many lacked media hardware or media savvy, and they were deprived even of this outlet.

As the numbers of dead and details of the pandemic dominated the media, and one's own life changed drastically, denial was impossible. Yet people needed mental relief. The most common means was disconnection. This could involve external withdrawal, or mental detachment and emotional numbness.

These disconnections themselves carried costs. People felt detached and empty, their minds were fuzzy, dizzy, and the world or oneself felt unreal. What was disconnected was sometimes felt physically or expressed behaviourally.

Common physical symptoms were dizziness, palpitations, shakes, choking in the throat and chest, nausea, frequency, diarrhoea, and pains in the head, neck, chest and back. Children were likely to express their distress in physical symptoms and behaviour.

Common behavioural changes included withdrawal, irritability, outbursts of anger and crying, overeating, drinking more alcohol, and immersion in the media, including gambling and sex.

One common and puzzling symptom, considering people were doing less, was fatigue. In part this was due to having to reassess every action that was previously automatic and effortless. Further, it took energy to maintain disconnections and to suppress tensions and emotions, and as the pandemic dragged on, frustration and despair sapped enthusiasm and energy.

As the pandemic continued, mental horizons, concentration and memory constricted. 'What did I come here for?' Time both dragged and flew. At other times reality burst through and feelings erupted, sometimes from a nightmare.

Cushioning against threatening appraisals carried short term benefits but also unnecessary costs.

An elderly lady was overwhelmed by leaden yet twisting heaviness in her chest and by her accompanying fatigue. Crying for what the pandemic had wrought in her life relieved both the heaviness and fatigue, but left her with full knowledge of her losses.

Ripples of the pandemic could become groundswells among the vulnerable.

The vulnerable

Stress was greater for the elderly, migrants, those in overcrowded housing, and those who had to work and could not keep social distancing. Fatal outbreaks occurred in social housing, abattoirs, retirement and nursing homes and in hospitals.

Children and adolescents, though relatively protected from the virus, were bored and missed school and friends. Some became withdrawn, obsessed with worries, and were moody, needy, angry, and teary. Their worlds, too, were turned upside down, and their parents, their protective buffers, became more unpredictable.

The **Already Stressed and Strained** were vulnerable to mental health issues especially if current circumstances fed into their vulnerabilities.

The following are disguised excerpts from a shared internet platform of a counselling service.

An anxiety has surfaced that I think was always there … I have taken up relaxation and exercise, which help me to stay together … I am overwhelmed, obsessed … My father works in a warehouse. What if he brings the virus home, especially to my immunosuppressed brother? … I shut off from it all. Sometimes ignorance is bliss … My partner can burst out in anger at me for no reason … I don't know what to do with all my feelings … Keeping busy helps me … I was made redundant. I am extremely sad … On top of my problems I have to bear my husband's emotional tornadoes… I feel rage at those who don't follow the rules … Families are breaking up all around … I just feel so powerless … I can't find any sort of happiness … I feel trapped and controlled …

Most of these people were not psychiatrically ill, but

they suffered a great variety of distressing mental health symptoms. They make emotional sense, but at the moment they are hard to classify, just like the earlier maelstrom of responses with which I started this book.

Sometimes aspects of the pandemic triggered specific past traumas. For instance, some Holocaust survivors entered states of anxiety and panic, which they associated with their pasts. For instance, lockdowns with police patrolling the streets triggered experiences of hiding with Nazis outside their homes.

Sometimes overt psychiatric illnesses were triggered by aspects of the pandemic. Cases like that accounted for the slight increase in overt psychiatric illnesses in the pandemic.

Andrew, 47, specialist in oceanography

Andrew had been severely abused as a child. Though currently a respected world expert in his profession, he nevertheless suffered severe social anxieties, relationship problems, and occasional paranoid psychotic episodes.

Because of the high rates of infection and death around him, he left America for his home in Melbourne. However, after his mandatory quarantine, a second wave of the virus broke out in Melbourne, and he had to go into lockdown.

Andrew felt persecuted and he entered a state of panic and paranoia.

Hospital staff were vulnerable to infection and to the stress and strain of looking after patients, many of whom died. Many staff members succumbed to the virus, or to burn-out.

Communities. For some already strained communities the pandemic was the last straw. For instance, in South Side Chicago, which had experienced racial inequality, government neglect, police brutality, gang warfare, and the recent televised death of George Floyd while under a white policeman's boot, Covid brought protests and violence to a new level. A resident reported more and more gunshots each night.

Paradoxically, some people improved in the pandemic. For instance some sufferers of agoraphobia who had not ventured outside their homes without severe anxiety, felt more comfortable as the rest of the population had to stay indoors.

How do we make sense of the myriad pictures of the pandemic?

There are so many stories. Everyone has a story. Those who died of the virus, their relatives, their doctors and carers; the ones in quarantine, those in lockdown, those awaiting disaster and those who recovered from it; parents and children; old, and young; families, groups, and nations; each has story and each story progresses from beginning, to middle, and end.

Each mind and combination of minds wobbles and struggles differently, each heart beats and sorrows at its own pace and feeling. And yet we are all limited within our skins.

So far the experiences and stories involve us, capture us. But sooner or later we must think about them and make sense of them in order to move stories to better places.

Imagine a child conveying that it is not well. We try to find words to refine the 'unwellnesses'. There is a tummy pain, headache, feeling like vomiting. We try to treat them, initially not realising that there are various reasons for each symptom. In time we have medical books and various specialties that refine unwellness and illnesses.

Unfortunately, medical and psychiatric books help only little in diagnosing the gamut of mental distress we have found so far.

In the pandemic we are at the stage of tummy pain, headache, and nausea. Their mental health equivalents, continually repeated, are suicide, anxiety, and depression.

We need a framework for the variety of symptoms we have encountered thus far.

The Wholist Framework

I intimated that there might be a kind of formula, a scientific perspective that can tether and make sense of the gamut of pandemic responses we have encountered so far. I foreshadowed that eight survival drives in three dimensions might present such a framework (a wholist framework).

Let us look at the three dimensions first.

Three Dimensions of the Pandemic

1. The Parameters Dimension. This dimension denotes the nature and context of the disaster. It orientates the *'what'* (in this case the pandemic), *'when'* it occurred, spread and ended, *'where'* it occurred, and *'who'* was affected: adults and children; individuals, families, community, nations, and the vulnerable and helpers.

The parameters axis is the scaffolding, or skeleton on which the flesh and blood of the pandemic is built.

2. The Process Dimension. This dimension denotes the progression of the pandemic from appraisals of means of survival through evoking survival drives, to their ripples and consequences. Survival drives (strategies) contain the apparently infinite and chaotic physical, psychological and social responses described thus far.

3. The Spiritual or Depth Dimension. This dimension is a specifically human one. It ranges from instincts to existential meanings and purpose. It includes morals, values, ideologies, religions, wisdom and truth.

Frequently ignored by the healing professions, this dimension includes pains that frequently exceed physical ones. Think of guilts, shames, angers at injustice; moral dilemmas, principles, values, self-esteem, existential meanings and purpose – people are willing to die for them, or they may be eternally tortured by them. (Think of having to choose who will have a respirator; having to work at the risk of infecting one's family, and so on.)

The three dimensions are depicted in Figure 1 below.

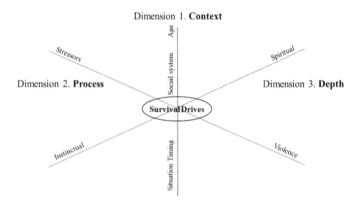

Dimension 1. **Context**

Context dimension	Process dimension	Depth dimension
1. Circumstances	1. Agonistic drives	1. Agonistic drives
2. Age	2. Evolutionary time	2. Morality
3. Social system	3. Traumatic time	3. Values and rights
4. Time	4. Current violence	4. Awe and sacredness
5. Place	5. Secondary spirals	5. Religions and ideologies
6. Person	6. Transgenerational	6. Meaning, purpose

It is impossible to keep the parameter, process, and spiritual dimensions in mind at the same time. Yet each point on each dimension is important. Like in medicine, missing out even one point can have tragic results. For instance, in Melbourne missing out on proper care of the elderly in nursing homes led to many deaths of the residents, and a second wave of the pandemic throughout the city.

Often children are forgotten. Often spiritual dilemmas are ignored.

Like in medicine eventually every system and organ must be considered, so in the pandemic we must sweep across its every possible dimension.

Survival Instincts. Survival Strategies

Survival instincts (often called survival drives or survival strategies) are the flesh and blood that cover and circulate through our three-dimensional framework.

Each survival strategy has biological, psychological, and social features, and they all have different nuances at different points of each dimension. This provides the impression of an infinity of responses. Yet all these responses can be traced back to one or other survival strategy evoked in specific threatening situations. Thus, we can potentially make sense of every symptom.

Alternatively, we can think of survival strategies as an octave, whose notes, with their harmonics and overtones can constitute complex symphonies; but each part of the symphony can be traced back to the original octave.

The octave of survival strategies is depicted in Table 1.

Table 1 Survival Drives

Appraisal of Means of Survival	Survival Drive	Anatomical Substrate	Adaptive / Coping Responses		
			biological	psychological	social
1. must save others	**rescue** protect provide	thalamus cingulate gyrus	↑estrogen ↑oxytocin ↑opioids	care empathy devotion	responsibility nurture preservation
2. must be saved by others	**attachment** protected provided	hypothalamus cingulate gyrus	?↑opioids	held cared for nutured looked after	close secure content union
3. must achieve goal	**achieve goal** combat work	hypothalamus lateral tegmentum	↑e, ↑ne ↓cortisol ↑immunocomp	strength control potency	will high morale success
4. must surrender goal	**adaptation** accept grieve	hippocampus septum	↑trophotropic ↑pit-adrenoc ↑cortisol	acceptance sadness grief hope	yielding mourning turning to new
5. must remove danger	**fight** defence	hypothalamus med-tegmentum amygdala	↑ne, renin, e ↑pit-adrenoc ↑cortisol	threat revenge frighten	deterrence wounding riddance
6. must remove oneself from danger	**flight** run hide save oneself	hypothalamus amygdala cingulate	↑erg & troph ↑da, b-end ?↑serotonin	fear terror deliverance	retreat flight escape
7. must obtain scarce essentials	**competition** dominance acquisition	hypothalamus hippocampus septum	↑testosterone ↑ne & e	winning status power	contest hierarchy possession
8. must create more essentials	**cooperation** trust mutual gain	amygdala temporal & cingulate gyri	↑opiates ↓bp, e & ne ↑trophotropic	mutuality generosity love	integration reciprocity creativity

Maladaptive / Not Coping Responses					Trauma Responses
*judgments of worth	biological	psychological	social	*judgments of worth	
responsible giving altruistic	ergotropic & trophotropic arousal	burden depletion self-concern	resentment neglect rejection	irresponsible neglectful egotistic	anguished compassion fatigue caused death
worthy deserving lovable	↓opioids ↑crf	yearning need craving abandonment	cling insecure deprived separation	unworthy encumberance rejectable	helplessness cast out left to die
strong capable successful	↑↑ergotropic ne depletion ↑bp, ?↑chd	frustration loss of control impotence	willfulness low morale failure	inadequate incompetent failure	exhaustion burn-out powerlessness
pitiful sympathy tribute	↑cortisol ↓immunocomp ↑infection?↑ca	overwhelmed depression despair	collapsed withdrawal giving-up	weak pathetic despicable	damaged given-in succumbing
brave nobel heroic	↑↑ergotropic arousal opioids vary ↓cort	hatred persecution killing	attack eradication destruction	violen wicked murderer	horror evil murder
pitiable vulnerable refugee	ne & da depletion ↑e & ↓cortisol	phobia paranoia engulfment	avoidance panic annihilation	timid panicky coward	inescapable shock being hunted, killed
superioir respected honored	↓testosterone ↓fsh & lh ↑acth	defeat greed envy exploitation	oppression struggle plunder	inferior contemptible humiliated	terrorization marginalization elimination
tender poignant beautiful	↓opiates ?trophotropic overactivity	betrayal selfishness abuse	disconnection robbery fragmentation	deceived seduced perverted	disintegration alienation decay

E, epinephrine; ne, norepinephrine; immunocomp, immunocompetence; pit-adrenoc, pituitary-adrenocortical axis; erg, ergotrophic system (arousal system including sympathetic nervous system); troph, trophotropic system (relaxation system including parasympathetic nervous system); bp, blood pressure; da, dopamine; b-end, beta endorphin; crf, corticotropin releasing factor; chd, coronary heart disease; ca, cancer; fsh, follicle stimulating hormone; lh, luteinising hormone; acth, adrenocorticotropic hormone.

The left half of the Table shows the fulfilling functions of survival strategies. The right side of the Table indicates the stresses, strains and traumas of stretched and overstretched survival strategies. The biological, psychological, and social aspects of these survival drives, as they radiate over three dimensions, constitute the myriad symptoms within stress and trauma situations such as the pandemic.

To add to (or elucidate) the complexity, survival strategies fluctuate according to circumstances, act in concert in various combinations, and vacillate between working and producing relief, or not working and causing symptoms.

Survival strategies can flare up in milliseconds from the instinctive, non-self-aware right hemisphere of the brain. People say, 'I did it automatically.' 'I was surprised that I had done that.' 'I didn't know that I could do it.'

Because much survival activity stems from the self-unaware right hemisphere, aspects of the survival activity make no sense and are experienced as mysterious symptoms.

Let us now look at such symptoms, previously encountered in a helter-skelter way, according to survival drives from which they originated. By simultaneously experiencing, as well as observing, orienting, naming, and understanding symptoms, we achieve a wholist perspective.

Rescue. Saving Others

It may come as a surprise that the first salient response in the pandemic, as in other disasters, was not dog eat dog or survival of the fittest, but the fittest attempting to save the weak and vulnerable. This was a strong instinct, manifest in parents protecting their children, health workers protecting patients, employers protecting their staff, and national leaders protecting their citizens (once it sank in that the corona virus could wipe out hundreds of thousands of them).

Saving lives became paramount. Sacrifices were made. Major changes occurred almost as a matter of fact. Opposition parties were enlisted to help. Facts and science overcame prior myths and ideologies. For instance, as intimated, in Australia, where for a conservative government a budgetary surplus was a sacred goal, within days the government somersaulted into a quasi-welfare state. In order to feed and support those who have been stood down and were unemployed and forced into idleness, the government incurred a debt not seen since the Second World War.

Health services that had been straining at the seams, were almost overnight allocated funds for staff, beds, respirators, and personal protective equipment.

At the coalface, the rescue instinct was intense and naked. We saw Laura who had to resist her drive to throw herself protectively on Mattia. The instinct usually radiated in the flesh and blood (or hearts and souls) in carers.

Nurse Natasha said, 'It is a massive privilege to be part of the health system. I am grateful that I can work and help people. It gives me purpose.'

Natasha's father, a devoted doctor, had died recently. She became teary, 'If my father was alive and capable, he wouldn't stop helping.' To renege her role would have betrayed him, her colleagues, her own values, and her sacred mission.

Stress on health care staff was enormous. They suffered anguish as their patients died. They were racked by guilt for having to choose who should live and die, like doctors had to in Italy. Staff suffered compassion fatigue, marked by exhaustion yet sleeplessness, and numbing of emotions yet underlying anguish.

Staff was constantly fearful of becoming infected and infecting patients and their families. By August in Victoria, in fact one third of infected cases were health care workers. This put more stress on the remaining staff.

Attachment: Seeking Rescue

Attachment is the other side of rescuing and saving. The rescuer's impulse to embrace is reciprocated by the impulse to hang on and cling by the rescued. Hugging and clinging form a secure, contented duo, exemplified between mother and baby or say, fire rescuer and the rescued.

As against disasters such as bushfires where rescuers

and rescued, and communities generally came together, the pandemic required separation and isolation. Signs everywhere indicated the 1.5 metres required between individuals. Handshakes were forbidden and were replaced by elbow rubs. Public places, restaurants, sports venues were all shut down or were severely restricted. The slogan, 'We're all in this together,' rang hollow.

Even at home the infected were isolated from their families and in hospitals carers wore distancing personal protective equipment, while the ill were covered in plastic tents (see Tony [p. 26] and Laura [p. 29]).

Many were lonely, as their yearning and need for others and their touch was unsatisfied. Many died alone and distressed. Relatives blocked from the sick and dying mirrored the distress.

Isolation and separations were ubiquitous. Workers were separated from work. Teenagers and young adults were separated from peers and romantic partners. For many children separation from school, teachers, and especially friends was the worst part of the pandemic. Internet connections could not replace physical proximity. Internet sex increased but was was devoid of reality. Many relationships suffered from separations.

In spite of this, many psychological attachments held. At home, children arranged their minds to changed relationships and parental directives. Similarly, adults absorbed the listened to authorities' pronouncements and imposed rules.

As noted, within days people gave up rights for which they had struggled for centuries: the right to movement, association, labour, even dress. Akin to the government somersaulting their ideologies, the population somersaulted from a democracy to a welfare police state.

What mattered was not prior ideologies or even religious beliefs, but current trust in the government and its intent to realistically protect its people.

Where leaders were incompetent or selfish, their nations were like dysfunctional families. Some followed their leaders, to their misfortune, while others, like orphaned children, struggled to be safe on their own.

For some the burdens were too great and they rebelled. Some young people had secret parties. Some diverted their frustrations into political protests, for instance claiming that their right to air was taken away. Some even rioted.

Goal Achievement. Hunting, Combat, Work

The virus thwarted everyday survival activities concerning food, security, shelter, and making things. The virus was an invisible army that needed to be hunted and combated out of existence.

So far we do not have the weapons to do that. We must await the vaccine on which our scientists are working. We scatter and hide until our weapons arrive.

Sometimes we stick our heads out, only to be hit

by another wave of casualties. Then we reluctantly, demoralised, retreat into our caves again.

Like soldiers forced into idle impotence while enemies lurk about, frustration sets in. Muscles tense, blood pressure rises. Macho men have to wait on women with test tubes to fight their battles and on the government to provide them with food.

Some rebel and express contempt for the enemy and those scared of it. They expose themselves, daring the enemy to attack them. Some divert aggression on weaker groups. But most do their best and try to occupy themselves in their fortresses.

Many could work from home, at least to some extent, but many could not. Some scraped what work they could. Others dipped into or emptied their superannuation funds or went into debt.

On a larger scale, economies slumped, businesses went broke, trade declined, and millions became unemployed. For the first time many depended on government handouts, charity, and soup kitchens. The conditions were compared to the Great Depression.

Many business owners and executives tried to adjust to ever-changing circumstances, which nevertheless were spiralling downhill. Many tried to support their employees with whom they had personal relationships. Many felt anguish having to fire employees in order to maintain their businesses.

Ted, aged 50, ran a large IT service with over 200 employees. The scene was ever-changing and deteriorating. Ted tried to keep the business afloat as it was losing millions each week. 'I have a heart, I know many employees and their families, but … it's simple maths. For the time being the government has come to our aid.'

Ted said with determination, 'I started this pandemic with 254 employees, and when it ends I will still have 254 employees.'

Many who still worked were vulnerable people and their work became more stressful. Some places of work like hospitals, abattoirs and warehouses became viral hotbeds.

Michael, aged 58 was an indigenous man who worked in a warehouse. Though grateful to have a job, he started to avoid his workmates some of whom, according to Michael, were not adhering sufficiently to COVID rules.

He himself tried to stay focused, do all the right things, and be self-disciplined, thus hoping to stay safe. Nevertheless, he was worried, slept poorly, and felt fatigued. 'I am disappointed, not on top of things. It's a hardy virus. I don't feel in control.'

Michael was urinating more frequently, indicating that his diabetes was out of control.

Government agencies suffered too. Public servants were made redundant. Quality of work suffered. All this while the government incurred unprecedented debt in order to prevent total chaos.

Everything became harder as outlets like libraries, sports venues, and restaurants closed.

Schools and universities closed too. Home schooling was challenging, and students worried about their exams and futures.

Morale kept falling. One's life hollowed. Self-image and dignity declined. One's view of oneself as a productive, contributing member of society suffered.

As always there were paradoxes. Some students worked better in isolation at home than they did at school. Some adults too, achieved more working at home than commuting for hours to offices. Some gained time for family recreations.

Adaptation. Goal Surrender. Loss

Humans are a very adaptable species, and it was remarkable how quickly people adjusted into the day-to-day requirements of surviving the pandemic.

It was unreal how routines that were the sinews of people's lives became dim memories. New views and perspectives were adopted like a change of clothes.

This picture was deceptive. The changes seemed unreal, even comic. But these were cushions from excessive pain. Actually people were shocked and stunned to different degrees by their new worlds.

Underneath the swift adaptation was hurtful loss. Most wounded were the ill, the dying, and the bereaved, especially when they had to say their goodbyes from afar.

Apart from bereavement, intimate contact between family members and close friends was often lost to different degrees. Michael (p. 48) wept because he couldn't comfort his two teenage children during the lockdown as they lived with his ex-wife in another state.

Losses were ubiquitous in the pandemic and every area was involved: relationships, work, school, routines, ways of life, enjoyments, and creativity; in a way the whole world had changed. Sometimes losses accrued. Sometimes they were additions to previous losses.

As in many other situations, people tried to cushion themselves against sadness and grief. But unexpressed grief and depression took a toll on physical and mental health.

Expressing bottled-up grief and despair could help.

Jane, 83, living with husband. As the second lockdown entered its third week, Jane became increasingly listless, and she lacked interest and energy. 'My legs feel like lead, and the heaviness goes up takes over my whole body. My chest feels heavy too, yet tight and painful. I'm so weighed down, that if I lie down, I might never get up, and anyhow, there is no point in getting up.'

What was the point, Jane explained. She hardly saw her children and grandchildren. Family gatherings, the sense of togetherness were gone. No birthday celebrations, no visits. She couldn't socialise with friends, couldn't do her hydrotherapy, art classes, visits to hairdresser; and all she hears is the number of infections and deaths.

Jane started to cry. Pangs of grief and sorrow were followed by deep sobs.

After she settled, she felt lighter. 'Love is still alive,' she said to her husband, 'and all this will be over some time too.'

Children's feelings and moods were influenced by parents' moods and directions. However, children of all ages felt losses and responded to them in their own way. Even children as young as two could be depressed and listless. However, children's lack of concentration and distractibility could obscure their depressions and their being overwhelmed.

It was clear that much was lost to the population and much would have to be grieved. But there was hope at the end of the tunnel. Perhaps a new, better world would emerge.

Fight

Fight is a hot-blooded kill or be killed instinctual drive. Fight is not a viable strategy against this pervasive invisible virus. No matter how much we hate it, we cannot engage and kill it. We must wait for the laborious technicians to provide the vaccine.

There is one exception and it occurs at the cellular level. Aided by high temperature of the blood (here we are hot-blooded), our immune system does fight the virus. An army of lymphocytes, macrophages and natural killer cells, engages, disables, poisons and ingests the opposing army of corona cells. This genocidal battle to the death goes on in infected individuals and is reflected in their clinical states.

Back on the macroscopic level, having to keep distance and isolate oneself from others tends to facilitate a view of others as potentially threatening. Individuals, families, neighbours, and groups have eyed each other warily as potentially risky. Endorsed by law, those infected were the most avoided. Those who tended them became suspect too. Sister Natasha (p. 44) was distressed because people hurled abuse at nurses who left the hospital in their uniforms.

The virus was associated with dirt. One had to frequently wash one's hands as if they were dirty. Disinfection was called deep cleaning. Boundaries formed between the clean and the dirty, between *us* and *them*, which could be defined by geography, nationality, ethnicity, race or economic status. Graffiti appeared calling on foreigners to go home. Borders between nations, states and districts solidified. Paranoia reached levels of enmity. Incidents of racism or social antipathy increased.

Let us be clear. The current pandemic has not elicited anything like the blaming of Jews for the Black Death pandemic in the 1300s, when thousands of Jews were burnt to death. But the corona virus has elicited frustrations, irritability and anger, which have translated into increased violence in the home and protests and riots, such as in the USA and Israel. But even in these cases there were factors outside the virus that were primary sources of anger.

These days we know that outsiders and even the infected are not dirty, and we recognise, for example, that underprivileged groups, which cannot afford to isolate and not work, do not deserve blame or guilt any more than health workers, who are infected at great rates.

Flight

Flight in the form of avoiding, distancing and hiding has been the most efficacious survival strategy available in the pandemic.

Associated emotions have included vigilance, fear, fright, terror and panic. When these emotions were suppressed, people felt a general anxiety. Fear and anxiety manifested in symptoms such as sleeplessness, nightmares, muscular tensions, trembling, butterflies in the stomach and need to void and defecate.

Fears of the virus could be displaced on to other fears, over which one may sense to have some control. Such fears included fear of going out (agoraphobia), obsessions such as constant washing of hands, or exaggerated concerns over slightest symptoms.

Fears and anxieties related to secondary effects of the

virus, such as unemployment, bankruptcy, and loss of residence, could be just as disabling as fear of the virus itself. These fears and anxieties could also be displaced onto phobias and obsessions. Prolonged fear is very taxing. Sometimes people 'rebel' and emerge, travel and congregate in spite of the consequences.

Anxieties and fears can trigger earlier anxieties and fears. For instance, when some Melbourne high rises experienced outbreaks of the virus, they were suddenly shut down and surrounded by police. Many residents were migrants who had experienced persecution. Like Holocaust survivors mentioned earlier, they were triggered back to feeling imprisoned and persecuted.

Children have also been fearful and anxious in different ways, according to their ages and parental behaviour. Some became clingy, others irritable. Others withdrew.

Parents and authorities need to try to modulate fears in their realms of responsibility, according to reality. Over-fear can lead to downward spirals of disabilities, while under-fear can lead to unwise behaviour, which in some instances can lead to contracting and spreading the disease.

Some people dealt with their fears and anxieties in creative ways. For instance, residents in the high rises who were shut down by police came together as never before, ignoring national and tribal differences. They established social media connections among themselves and with the police, who soon withdrew.

Competition. Struggle

Television-displayed struggles for food and toilet rolls in supermarkets epitomised competition for what were perceived to be looming scarcities.

On a more serious level, hospitals, states, and nations struggled for supplies of beds, masks, gowns, personal protective equipment, and respirators. Scarce beds and respirators meant, as happened in Cremona, that some patients had to be chosen for treatment over others.

On national levels, China bought up emergency equipment from around the world at the start of the pandemic. In the USA, President Trump promoted hydroxychloroquine in the belief that Americans would preferentially benefit from its supposed anti-Covid–19 activity. Laboratories around the world raced to be the first to discover a vaccine. Their citizens would be the first to benefit.

These were transparent competitive actions. But there was a more entrenched, covert, more widespread competition: between the rich and powerful and the poor and powerless. This competition was relatively invisible because it took place according to long established hierarchies.

The result of this inequality showed in poorer people having higher rates of corona infections and deaths. For instance, in the USA black and indigenous people died from the virus at twice the rate of whites. Differential infection and mortality rates occurred also in previous pandemics. Actually the wealthy generally have better health than the poor.

In the pandemic the wealthy already started with better health and access to treatments. They were able to evacuate to sparsely populated holiday homes, or could batten down in comfortable spacious homes with plentiful access to resources. Poorer individuals and nations started the pandemic in physically, mentally and socially compromised circumstances. They had to live in crowded conditions, and had to work in menial, sometimes dangerous jobs.

Overlapping with the poor, other sections of the community also fared worse than others. They included the ill, the disabled, the elderly (especially those in deprived, poorly run nursing homes), the isolated, migrants, asylum seekers, temporary visa holders, and students. Many slid down the social scale and joined the ranks of the vulnerable following losing their jobs.

In addition to physical hazards of infection, the poor and the vulnerable often suffered powerlessness, defeat, and loss of self-esteem and identity. They suffered moral injury. A man on a temporary visa felt 'wronged and without any support after five years paying my taxes and being part of the community'. Another said, 'The Australian government treated people on working holiday visas as consumable.'

Sometimes demeaned men asserted themselves aggressively, even violently, in domestic violence or in the community. However, on the whole, this was rare. Governments, such as the Australian one, provided financial grants to the poor and grants to employers to keep jobs open. This maintained a supply of goods and avoided dog eat dog social chaos. Rather than struggling as for toilet rolls, as depicted on TV, people queued quietly for food and essentials.

At the top end of the hierarchical scale, some rationalised that it was their evolutionary right to behave as they wished as they were the preferred ones in nature's survival of the fittest. Some donated a little of their wealth to appease their guilt.

Much more commonly the better off donated money and their services to the poor. Some were extremely generous. And some nations promised that the vaccine, when it arrived, would be justly and evenly distributed to everyone around the world.

Cooperation. Creativity

'We're all in this together!' has been a common catchcry, and indeed, uniquely, everyone in the world has been threatened with the corona virus.

In the face of a common enemy people did come together. Families, together for more time, intensified their relationships. Neighbours who had little in common before offered help to each other. Indigenous people from different tribes formed common 'mobs'. Especially initially, when the length of the pandemic was not appreciated, there was a wave of euphoria as from politicians down to individuals people put aside their differences and merged in a common cause.

There was optimism that this solidarity would continue to translate into common purpose and past divisions and enmities would be forgotten. It seemed that if we could cooperate on the virus, we could cooperate on climate change, on nuclear weapons, on poverty.

It is said, 'Necessity is the mother of invention.' Of course the invention we all want is the vaccine, but in the meantime individuals and societies invented new ways to live, work, trade, communicate, learn, enjoy, make things, and create. Some of these inventions would provide permanent benefits.

Euphoria, cooperation and creativity are common at the beginning of wars and other challenges. In the beginning a quick victory is anticipated. But this war has dragged on. Cooperation in the second wave was through gritted teeth rather than euphoria. Some faltered to cooperate.

Forced togetherness could be irritating and fraying. Stress can reduce creativity, libido and tolerance. Families have broken up during the pandemic. But love flourishes after disasters and birth rates increase.

Much will depend on future leaderships as to which survival strategies will reign. Hopefully, it will be less competition and fight, and more cooperation and creativity.

Diagnosis Of Pandemic Stress Responses

For a long time, each survival strategy was recognised, but the octave has not been assembled to explain the great variety of symptoms in stressful and traumatic situations.

This has led to a constriction of our language. For instance, we may use the term 'depression' for sadness, grief, fatigue, defeat, loneliness, failure, demoralisation, and so on, without realising that each belongs to specific still undefined areas. The same is true for 'anxiety', which may cover concepts of causing harm, being abandoned, being harmed, betrayed, and so on. Even suicidal ideas may arise not only from 'depression', but also from anguish, guilt, shame, injustice, failed values and ideals, arising from failed survival strategies.

Awareness of survival strategies provides us with a vocabulary that recognises previously inchoate 'mental health consequences' of disasters, previously limited by language to suicide rates, anxiety, and depression.

The wholist perspective enables us to orientate and make sense of the great variety of survival strategy responses, be they physical, psychological, social or spiritual.

Dealing With Mental Health Consequences of the Pandemic

Treatment regimes go by many names, but certain elements apply to mental health treatments in all disasters, including the pandemic.

Recognition

It was important to recognise the nature, extent and danger of the pandemic in order to manage it realistically. Without recognition one is subject to denial, over-fear, rumours, myths and fantasies, but worst of all, one is vulnerable to the ravages of the virus.

Authorities needed to be truthful and caring in order to be believed and their instructions to be followed. In Australia the government, with scientists by their sides, earned the population's trust as they provided their daily updates and instructions.

Similarly, people generally trusted government information in newspapers, on radio, television, electronic media, and in publications.

Official recognition of mental health consequences of the disaster took a little longer, even though workers in the field clamoured for resources as they were faced with increased numbers of people seeking help.

Education. Advice. Counselling

Once recognised, treatments were instituted. The first and commonest line of treatment was supportive. It included education, advice and counselling.

Education. People were advised of common responses to crises, such as in the pamphlet *Coping With a Major Personal Crisis* put out by the Red Cross (see chapter 2). A core message was *'Your distress is normal. It is the circumstances that are abnormal.'* People were not crazy and they need not feel shame about how they felt.

Advice. Advice included: establish routines of meals, diet, sleep, rest, exercise, and time out to rest and think; try to keep life as normal as possible; set and accomplish immediate goals; utilise modern media for work, learning, amusement and maintaining contacts; communicate and share with meaningful others; express your needs clearly and honestly to family, friends, officials, and mental health workers; do not bottle up feelings.

Counselling. Counselling included warnings and means of relief.

Warnings included: be extra careful with machinery and cars, because stress distracts and leads to accidents; maintain your usual medications; be wary of alcohol, non-prescribed drugs, gambling and overeating.

Techniques of tension and stress relief included deep

breathing, relaxation exercises, yoga, meditation, massage, hydrotherapy, and enjoying simple pleasures such as walks in nature.

All treatments accrue much benefit from human interaction. They were considered to be non-specific parts of treatment, but actually their ingredients have specific counter-stress effects.

Relationships. Counter Stress Ingredients

What applies to authorities regarding genuine care and trust applies also to professional carers and therapists. Their 'human' characteristics make their efforts credible and trusted. What they provide has these ingredients:

Sense **of a *safe trusted environment*—**whether in an office, or as was necessary in the pandemic, over the screen.

'Being there'; responding as a 'human' engenders trust and security.

Kindness, comforting and support enhance sense of importance and being worthwhile.

Empathy, being listened to, caring, holding, nurturing provide a sense of attunement and being understood.

Space and boundaries provide an area to think, talk, play, and work.

Non-judgemental attitudes and respect counter negative self-judgements.

Hope including good cheer, confidence, humour, and realistic positive expectations (glass half full) counter excessive pessimism and despair.

Symptomatic Treatments

Symptomatic treatments are aimed at removing symptoms without prime concern for insight for their origins. Examples are treating headaches and other pains with pain killers; stomach symptoms with antacids; anxiety with tranquilisers; sleeplessness with sleeping tablets; depression with anti-depressants.

Similarly, fears are treated with fear reduction (through gradual exposure to feared objects); anger with anger management; aloneness with facilitating contacts; financial problems are addressed by financial advisors; unemployment with employment agencies, and so on.

These are all supportive treatments in which both clients and helpers are aware of the logic of the help that is provided.

Some symptoms persist and do not make sense. That is because they symbolise deep problems, which people sense, if exposed, could destroy their lives. In this case, supportive therapy must be expanded into insight therapy.

A wide range of therapies focus on specific symptoms. They include cognitive behaviour therapy (CBT), eye movement and desensitisation and reprocessing therapy (EMDR), and focal psychotherapy.

What they all have in common is recognition of the symptom as symbolic of a past highly stressful or traumatic situation, which the person could not resolve at the time. In that situation the client had done his or her best, but the situation was too overwhelming and painful. That situation is now in the past, though it is imprinted on the mind as if it was still current. With increasing clarity the conditions of the past trauma and current safety are separated and imbued with distance of time and narrative meaning.

Treatment Within a Wholist Perspective

When a person survives a severe car crash he or she needs a through physical examination. Each area of the body, each organ and system is looked at and assessed in depth. Everything around the circumstances and consequences of the crash must be attended to.

The same multidimensional approach must be applied to mental health consequences of disasters like the pandemic.

The wholist perspective includes all the elements of treatment considered thus far: recognition, education, relationship, and symptom reduction.

But when everything is up in the air, catching one problem is only an opportunity for another problem to emerge. Just as following a car crash we wouldn't stop with appeasing one symptom or issue of the event, so we cannot be satisfied with appeasing one mental health symptom such as anxiety or depression, suicidal thoughts or domestic violence; especially now that our eyes have been opened to so many other symptoms in different dimensions that occur in stress and trauma.

Remember the stone in the pond? It causes multiple ripples across the length, breadth and depth of the pond. A major disturbance like a pandemic causes a variety of ripples across every dimension. Dealing with one ripple, or even progression of a ripple, is insufficient. A major disturbance disturbs the whole. We need a wholist perspective.

At the very least we need to find an epicentre, the central disturbance of the stone hitting the water, the moment of collision of two cars, the initial infection of the virus. We can then sweep over the multiple ripples. Or, when the collision is not remembered, we may trace the ripples back to its epicentre.

Just like every human has similar features but is different in detail, so all pandemic pictures are tethered to the wholist perspective and can be examined through it

Among the millions of such pictures let us briefly look at Laura (pp. 28-30) as a brief example.

Were you to seek out the epicentre of her distress and ask 'Of all the things that worry you, what worries you the most?' she might say that it was having had to choose whom to intubate and whom to leave to die. Her rescue instinct was traumatised but still alive when she wanted to embrace the boy who was afraid of dying. Her other instincts were overstretched. She was in combat in 12-hour shifts but no matter how much energy she expended she could not succeed. She felt defeated competing for scarce resources. She couldn't fight the virus. 'We're dropping like flies.' And eventually she succumbs to the virus. She becomes dependent on others. She recalls all the dead. There were too many to grieve. She has suicidal ideas.

Her symptoms relate to the gamut of overstretched survival strategies (Table 1). Were we to treat Laura, in the context of the therapeutic relationship (see other treatment elements) we would recognise, name, talk about, trace to its origins, re-feel, reassess, put in context, process, and place her traumas in a self-aware forgiving, moral, existential framework, now in her power. A similar process may be required for her family, and her colleagues.

All survival strategies in all their dimensions are to be covered. Helping professionals may demur, saying that they are not trained to heal the variety of biological, psychological and social problems. Further, they do not have time to cover the whole human condition of their clients. Yet it is not too difficult to learn how different survival strategies manifest in their different guises. In fact, a wholist perspective saves time, just like recognizing and dealing with all current physical disturbances does in general medicine.

In practice, factors of recognition and insight, counselling, counter-stress relationships and wholist treatments combine. The wholist perspective ensures that a wide variety of symptoms can be understood in their contexts and receive appropriate treatments.

That is the purpose of this booklet: to convert painful experiences into understandable stories that make sense and heal. This is not a luxury perspective. Missing out on aspects of it can have dire consequences. Including them can restore love and soul into our shaken selves.

References

Australian Red Cross. *Coping with a Major Personal Crisis* (pamphlet).

Emergency Management Australia (2002). *Mental Health Practitioners Guide.*

Valent, P. (1998). *From Survival to Fulfilment*; *A Framework for the Life–Trauma Dialectic*. London: Taylor and Francis.

Valent, P. (1998). *Trauma and Fulfilment Therapy*; *A Wholist Framework*. London: Taylor and Francis.

Printed in Australia
AUHW011003041120
336597AU00010B/28